I0698122

Table of Contents

Gallstones are hardened deposits of digestive fluid that can form in your gallbladder. Your gallbladder is a small, pear-shaped organ on the right side of your abdomen, just beneath your liver. The gallbladder holds a digestive fluid called bile that's released into your small intestine.

Gallstones range in size from as small as a grain of sand to as large as a golf ball. Some people develop just one gallstone, while others develop many gallstones at the same time.

People who experience symptoms from their gallstones usually require gallbladder removal surgery. Gallstones that don't cause any signs and symptoms typically don't need treatment.

BREAKFAST

1. Roasted Winter Veggie Gnocchi

Prep Time: 10 Minutes

Cook Time: 20 Minutes

Servings: 4

Ingredients

- 1 red onion in 1/2" pieces
- 1 butternut squash in 1/2" pieces
- 2 parsnips in 1/2" pieces
- 2 cups brussels sprouts quartered
- 2 garlic cloves sliced
- 1 tablespoon olive oil
- 1 tablespoon sage chopped
- 1/2 pound gnocchi
- 1 cup spinach chopped
- 2 tablespoon olive oil
- 1 tablespoon lemon juice
- 1 teaspoon sage chopped

- 1 teaspoon thyme chopped
- 1/4 cup parmesan grated
- 1/4 cup walnuts chopped

Instructions

1. Preheat oven to 400 degrees Fahrenheit.
2. Toss red onion, butternut squash, parsnips, Brussels sprouts, and garlic with olive oil and sage.
3. Roast for 15-20 minutes.
4. Meanwhile, boil a large pot of water.
5. When veggies are done, pour gnocchi into the boiling water and cook for 2-3 minutes or until they are all floating.
6. Drain, reserving about 1/4 cup of pasta water, and return to the pot. Add veggies and the rest of the ingredients as well as the pasta water.
7. Mix well, top with walnuts, and enjoy!

Prep Time: 5 Minutes

Cook Time: 15 Minutes

Servings: 4

Ingredients

- 8 ounces whole wheat penne pasta
- 2 tablespoons extra virgin olive oil
- 3 garlic cloves minced
- 1/2 teaspoon red chili flakes
- 1 pound shrimp deveined, peeled, tails removed
- Salt to taste
- Black pepper to taste
- 2 cups brown mushrooms sliced
- 1 lemon juiced
- 1/4 cup parsley plus 2 tablespoons, fresh, chopped
- 1/4 cup parmesan grated

Instructions

1. Cook the penne pasta until al dente. When the pasta is finished, drain it but reserve about 1/4 cup cooking water.
2. Meanwhile, in a large skillet, heat 1 tabelspoon olive oil on medium high heat.
3. Sauté garlic and chili flakes for about 1 minute.
4. Add shrimp and season with salt and pepper. Cook for about 2-3 minutes or until the shrimp turns pink.
5. Remove shrimp from the pan and add mushrooms, salt, pepper, and sauté for another 5 minutes.
6. Add the cooked pasta, shrimp, lemon juice, remaining olive oil, cooking water, parmesan, chopped parsley and toss over medium heat until well combined.
7. Garnish with remaining parsley and enjoy!

Prep Time: 10 Minutes

Cook Time: 30 Minutes

Servings: 4

Ingredients

- 1 tablespoon olive oil
- 3 cloves garlic minced
- 1/2 cup yellow onion diced small
- 18 ounces crimini mushrooms sliced
- 1 teaspoon kosher salt
- 1/3 cup white wine
- 1 tablespoon tamari sauce
- 2 tablespoons dark balsamic vinegar
- 1 tablespoon dijon mustard
- 1/2 cup coconut milk light
- 2/3 cup water

Instructions

1. In a large skillet, heat the olive oil. Once hot, add the garlic, onion, and mushrooms. Season with the salt.

Cook on medium for about 15 minutes or until onions are translucent and mushrooms are soft.

2. Stir in the white, simmer until the liquid is reduced by half. This can take around ten minutes.

3. Add the remaining ingredients. Simmer for about 20 minutes, stirring often, or until the mixture is thickened and reduced. Serve over mashed potatoes, gluten-free vegan pasta, quinoa, riced cauliflower, or any grain combined with greens.

Prep Time: 5 Minutes

Cook Time: 25 Minutes

Servings: 6

Ingredients

- 1 tablespoon olive oil
- 1 yellow onion diced
- 3 garlic cloves minced
- 1 cup carrots diced
- 1/2 cup celery diced
- 1 green bell pepper diced
- 1 cup zucchini diced
- 1 pound spicy Italian sausage
- 1 teaspoon mixed Italian herbs
- 1/2 teaspoon red chili flakes
- 1/2 teaspoon ground black pepper
- 13.5 ounces canned diced tomatoes
- 5 cups low sodium chicken broth
- 1 pound russet potatoes peeled and cut into 1/2" cubes
- 4 cups kale chopped

Instructions

1. Heat olive oil in a large pot over medium heat
2. Add onion, garlic, carrots, celery, green bell pepper, and zucchini and saute for 3 minutes
3. Add sausage and seasoning and cook for about 5 minutes, breaking up the sausage as you stir
4. Add diced tomatoes, black pepper, chicken broth, potatoes, and kale
5. Bring to a simmer for 15 minutes or until potatoes are tender

Prep Time: 10 Minutes

Cook Time: 20 Minutes

Servings: 6

Ingredients

- 8 ounces chickpea pasta we used Banza linguine
- 1.5 pound chicken breast boneless, skinless fillets
- 2 tablespoons Cajun blackening seasoning
- 4 tablespoons butter
- 2 garlic cloves minced
- 1 shallot minced
- 1 teaspoon dried mixed herbs
- Dash salt and pepper
- 1 cup milk
- 2 cups water
- 2 tablespoons cornstarch
- 1 cup parmesan cheese grated
- 1/4 cup parsley fresh, chopped

Instructions

1. Start by cooking the chickpea pasta according to package instructions.

2. Meanwhile, coat the chicken breasts with the Cajun blackened seasoning.

3. Heat a large cast-iron skillet on medium-high. Once hot, melt butter in the skillet.

4. When that has melted, add the seasoned chicken and cook for about 5 minutes per side or until cooked through.

5. Remove from heat. After letting it rest, slice into strips.

6. Get a new skillet or clean out your original one, put it over medium heat, and melt the other 2 tablespoons of butter.

7. Add garlic, shallot, mixed herbs, and salt and pepper for about 1 minute, then pour in the milk, water, and cornstarch and mix well.

8. Bring the heat down to low and let simmer for about 5 minutes or until thickened, then add the parmesan cheese and let it melt.

9. Add chicken and pasta and gently toss. Top with parsley and enjoy!

Prep Time: 5 Minutes

Cook Time: 30 Minutes

Servings: 4

Ingredients

- 3 cups chicken cooked, shredded
- 3 cups broccoli cut in florets
- 4 cups brown rice cooked
    - ounces light cream of mushroom soup canned
- 2 teaspoons curry powder
- 1 cup low-fat cheddar cheese shredded

Instructions

1. Combine all of the ingredients except for ¼ cup of cheddar cheese in a bowl, mixing well
2. Spread evenly into a greased 9 x 13 baking dish
3. Sprinkle the rest of the cheese over top, then cover with foil
4. Bake for 25 minutes, then uncover and bake for another 5 minutes.

5. Remove from the oven and let rest for about 5 minutes before serving

Prep Time: 20 Minutes

Cook Time: 1hr 10 Minutes

Servings: 6

Ingredients

- 1 tablespoon olive oil divided
- 2 teaspoons sea salt
- 2 eggplants sliced in thin rounds
- 1 garlic clove minced
- 2 cups brown mushrooms sliced
- 2 cups spinach chopped
- 3/4 cup low fat ricotta
- 1/4 cup parmesan cheese shredded
- 1 egg
- 1/2 tablespoon Italian herb seasoning
- 1 1/2 cup part-skim mozzarella cheese
- 32 oz marinara sauce
- 1/4 cup whole wheat bread crumbs
- 3 tablespoons parsley fresh, chopped

Instructions

1. Toss the eggplant rounds with ½ tbs of olive oil and salt, then lay evenly on a baking sheet
2. Bake in the oven for about 20 minutes or until soft and slightly golden, flipping halfway.
3. Meanwhile, heat the other 1⁄2 tablespoon of olive oil in a skillet over medium high heat.
4. Add the garlic for about 1 minute, and then toss in mushrooms. Saute for 4-5 minutes or until softened, then add spinach for another minute or so to wilt. Remove from heat.
5. In a medium bowl, mix together the low fat ricotta, parmesan, egg, and seasoning.
6. In a 9×13 baking dish, spread about ½ a cup of marinara sauce in the bottom of the pan, then lay a layer of eggplant (about ⅓ of the slices)
7. Top with ⅓ cup of the ricotta mixture, ⅓ of the mushrooms and spinach mix, and then ½ cup of mozzarella
8. Start a new layer with ¾ cup of marinara sauce and continue layering in this order until finished
9. Top the casserole with a sprinkle of breadcrumbs

10. Cover and bake at 400 degrees for about 45 minutes. Remove the foil and bake for 10 more minutes. Let cool, top with parsley, and enjoy!

Prep Time: 7 Minutes

Cook Time: 20 Minutes

Servings: 8

Ingredients

- 1 puff pastry
- 2 tablespoons olive oil extra virgin
- 4 tablespoons Parmesan grated
- 2 garlic cloves minced
- 1 teaspoon Italian seasoning blend
- 1 teaspoon kosher salt
- 1/4 teaspoon black pepper ground

Instructions

1. Preheat oven to 400F. Roll the puff pastry onto a baking sheet lined with parchment paper.
2. Add the remaining ingredients to a small bowl and mix until combined.
3. Spread the parmesan mixture onto the puff pastry. Then roll the puff pastry and cut it into 8 slices.

4. Bake for 15-20 minutes or until the puffs are golden
    brown.

Prep Time: 10 Minutes

Cook Time: 8hrs 3 Minutes

Servings: 16

Ingredients

- 2 tablespoons extra virgin olive oil
- 1 yellow onion diced
- 2 garlic cloves minced
- 1 tablespoon basil freshly chopped
- 1 teaspoon black pepper
- 2 pounds snap green beans fresh or frozen, rinsed and strings removed
- 1 potato medium, peeled and diced
- 3 cups vegetable broth or chicken broth, low-sodium, fat-free
- Kosher or sea salt to taste

Instructions

1. In a medium skillet saute onion and garlic on medium-low heat until tender, about 4 minutes. Add sauteed

onion and garlic along with all other ingredients to the slow cooker. Recommend 5-7 quart slow cooker.

2. Cover and cook on low 8 hours. Cooking time may vary depending on how tender you like your green beans. Southern-style green beans are typically cooked until they are falling apart.

Prep Time: 00 Minutes

Cook Time: 00 Minutes

Servings: 6

Ingredients

- 1 tablespoon olive oil
- 1 yellow onion chopped
- 2 garlic cloves minced
- 1 jalapeno pepper minced (optional)
- 1 tablespoon tomato paste
- 1 teaspoon ground cumin
- 1 tablespoon chili powder
- 3 cups vegetable broth low-sodium
- 15 ounces diced tomatoes can, no sugar added
- 15 ounces black beans can, low-sodium, drained and rinsed
- 15 ounces corn kernels can, low-sodium
- 4 corn tortillas 6 inch, cut into 1/2 inch strips

Instructions

1. Preheat the oven to 450 degrees.
2. Heat the olive oil in a large soup pot on medium heat, once hot add the onion, garlic, and jalapeno. Cook until the onions are soft, about 5 minutes. Stir in the tomato paste and cooking, stirring frequently, for one minute.
3. Stir in the cumin, chili powder, broth, tomatoes, beans, and corn. Mix well and bring to a simmer. Simmer for 15 minutes.
4. Meanwhile, spread half of the tortilla strips on a baking sheet. Bake for 5 to 10 minutes or just until crisp.
5. Stir in the remaining tortilla strips into the soup. Ladle into serving bowls and top with the crisp tortillas.

11. Clean Eating Chicken Salad

Prep Time: 15 Minutes

Cook Time: 00 Minutes

Servings: 4

Ingredients

- 2 boneless and skinless chicken breasts cooked, cut into cubes
- 2 celery stalks chopped
- 1/4 red onion chopped
- 1/2 cup red seedless grapes quartered
- 1/2 cup Greek yogurt non-fat
- 1 teaspoon garlic powder
- 1 teaspoon black pepper freshly ground
- Sea salt to taste
- 2 whole-wheat pita pockets halved
- 4 romaine lettuce

Instructions

1. In a large bowl, mix all of the salad ingredients. Chicken salad can be eaten as is or eat as a pita sandwich. Recipe serves 4.

Prep Time: 10 Minutes

Cook Time: 5 Minutes

Servings: 2

Ingredients

Creamy Tuna:

- 5 ounces chunk light tuna in water can, drained
- 1/4 cup Greek yogurt low-fat, plain or clean mayo
- 1/4 teaspoon kosher or sea salt
- 1/4 teaspoon black pepper

To Assemble:

- 4 butter lettuce leaves or iceberg, large
- 1 whole-wheat wrap large
- 1/2 cup cheddar cheese reduced-fat, shredded
- 4 pickle slices or jalapeño slices, optional

Instructions

2. Mix together all ingredients for creamy tuna. Spread in a broiler-safe baking dish/pan and sprinkle cheese on

top. Place under broiler for one to two minutes, just until cheese melts.

3. Lay wrap flat and line with lettuce leaves. Scoop tuna with melted cheese over wrap. Top with pickles or pickled jalapeño slices, if using. Tuck under one end and roll wrap. Cut in half and serve.

Prep Time: 10 Minutes

Cook Time: 00 Minutes

Servings: 2

Ingredients

- 2 slices multigrain bread
- 2 tablespoons roasted garlic hummus or hummus of choice
- 3 tomato slices
- 1/2 cup baby spinach
- 1/8 teaspoon salt a pinch sprinkled on

Instructions

1. Toast multigrain bread (if desired). Spread hummus on top of one slice of bread. Top with tomato slices and layer with spinach. Spinkle on salt. Place the second slice of bread on top. Serve and enjoy!

Prep Time: 15 Minutes

Cook Time: 15 Minutes

Servings: 6

Ingredients

- 1 tablespoon extra-virgin olive oil
- 2 garlic cloves minced
- 1 red onion small, cut in half and then thinly sliced
- 1 cup bell peppers sliced
- 1 zucchini small, sliced
- 1/2 cup pizza sauce (Skinny Ms. Recipe)
- 1/2 cup sun dried tomatoes diced or 2 Roma tomatoes, sliced
- 8 green olives diced
- 1 tablespoon fresh basil chopped
- 1/2 cup skim mozzarella cheese shredded
- 1 whole wheat thin pizza crust 10 or 12 inch

Instructions

2. Preheat oven to 450°.

3. In a large skillet, add oil, and sauté on medium-low heat for 1 minute, the garlic, onion, bell peppers (if using the Balsamic Bell Pepper recipe, do not sauté with the other ingredients), and zucchini slices.

4. Spread sauce over the crust, leaving 1 inch around the edges dry. Evenly distribute onto crust the garlic, onion, bell peppers, zucchini, sun-dried tomatoes, olives, basil, and mozzarella cheese. Preferably, place pizza directly onto middle oven rack. Otherwise, place pizza on a large cooking stone or cookie sheet. Bake 10 minutes or until cheese is melted and bubbly.

Prep Time: 15 Minutes

Cook Time: 25 Minutes

Servings: 9

Ingredients

- 1 pound lean ground beef optional ground turkey
- 1 onion small, diced
- 1/2 teaspoon sea salt
- 1/2 teaspoon black pepper
- 3 bell peppers medium, varied colors (remove core, seeds, and membrane)
- 2/3 cup ketchup divided
- 1 tablespoon mustard
- 5 slices cheddar cheese reduced-fat (any cheese will work)

Instructions

1. Preheat oven to 375 degrees.
2. Slice each bell pepper into 6 vertical pieces, along the indention line. Set peppers aside.

3. In a large mixing bowl combine meat, onion, salt, pepper, 1/3 cup ketchup, and mustard.

4. Add meat mixture to boats. Place on a parchment-lined baking sheet and cook until meat is done, about 20 minutes.

5. Remove boats from the oven, drizzle with remaining ketchup, then top each with 1/4 cheese slice, place back in the oven and bake just until cheese is melted, about 5 minutes.

6. Remove boats and enjoy will hot!

Prep Time: 5 Minutes

Cook Time: 3hrs 2 Minutes

Servings: 6

Ingredients

- 1 onion small, diced
- 1 celery stalk diced
- 2 carrots peeled and sliced
- 1 zucchini sliced
- 1 large potato peeled and cubed
- 2 cups green beans fresh or frozen
- 1 cup peas fresh or frozen
- 2 cups kale coarsely chopped or other green leafy vegetable like spinach or chard
- 2 cups vegetable broth or water (add 1 additional cup for a thinner minestrone)
- 15 ounces diced tomatoes can, with liquid
- 15 ounces kidney beans can, drained and rinsed
- 1/2 cup vegetable juice or tomato juice
- 1 teaspoon kosher or sea salt
- 1/4 teaspoon ground black pepper

- 4 basil leaves fresh, diced
- 1/2 cup parmigiano reggiano or parmesan

Instructions

1. Add all ingredients to a slow cooker, except kale, basil, and parmesan. Cover and cook on low 5 to 6 hours or high 3 to 4 hours.

2. When the minestrone is cooked, add kale. Place lid back on slow cooker and allow the kale to wilt, approximately 5 minutes.

3. When ready to serve the minestrone, drizzle a little extra-virgin olive oil over the top of individual bowls. Sprinkle with fresh basil and Parmigiano Reggiano or Parmesan.

4. Optional: Add 1 cup whole wheat penne pasta 30 minutes before the end of cooking.

Prep Time: 10 Minutes

Cook Time: 00 Minutes

Servings: 6

Ingredients

Salad:

- 6 cups romaine heart lettuce chopped
- 2 avocados ripe, seeded and peeled, slice into 1 inch pieces
- 1 split chicken breast cooked, skin removed and cubed
- 2 tomatoes vine-ripe, chopped
- 2 hard-boiled eggs peeled and sliced

Dressing:

- 1/4 cup red wine vinegar
- 1/2 cup extra virgin olive oil
- 1 teaspoon honey or maple syrup
- kosher or sea salt to taste
- 1/8 teaspoon black pepper

Instructions

1. Combine salad ingredients in a large bowl. Combine
   dressing ingredients and drizzle over salad.

Prep Time: 00 Minutes

Cook Time: 00 Minutes

Servings: 6

Ingredients

- 18 rice paper wrappers
- 8 ounces brown rice noodles recommend Annie Chun's Maifun Brown Rice Noodles
- 5 ounces mixed baby greens organic if possible
- 1 avocado
- 1 cucumber
- 2 bell peppers your choice of color
- 2 cups carrots shredded
- 2 cups purple cabbage shredded
- 16 ounces tofu firm or super firm
- Vegan oil-free salad dressing – your choice

Instructions

2. Prepare rice noodles according to package instructions and then drain.

3. Peel and slice avocado, cucumber, and bell peppers into matchstick width strips.

4. Prepare tofu planks as described in this recipe, without the marinade, and then slice into matchstick width strips.

5. Add the vegetable fillings to a large bowl, then toss and coat liberally with the vegan oil-free salad dressing of your choice.

6. Prepare rolls individually by submerging one sheet of rice wrapper at a time in a bowl of warm water for 10 seconds, then place on a cutting board or other clean, flat work surface.

7. Layer an even amount of salad filling across the lower third of the rice wrapper, leaving room on sides to tuck edges for your burrito spring rolls.

8. Layer an even amount of tofu strips and rice noodles over salad filling, then fold over edge flaps and roll your burritos into fully enclosed tubes.

9. The ingredients listed should make about 18 finished rolls. Place finished rolls on a serving tray, and be sure not to stack them, as they will stick together.

10. Eat, smile, and feel healthy!

Prep Time: 10 Minutes

Cook Time: 10 Minutes

Servings: 4

Ingredients

- 1/2 tablespoon olive oil
- 1 pound lean sirloin steak sliced into very thin strips
- 1/2 teaspoon kosher salt
- 1/4 teaspoon ground black pepper
- 2 teaspoons dry oregano leaves
- 1 yellow onion sliced into strips
- 1 green bell pepper sliced into strips
- 1 red bell pepper sliced into strips
- 8 lettuce leaves large, such as bibb lettuce
- 1/2 cup provolone cheese shredded (reduced-fat if available)
- 2 tablespoons cilantro fresh, roughly chopped

Instructions

1. In a large skillet on high heat, add the olive oil. Once hot, add the steak and season with salt and pepper. Add the oregano, onion, and the green and red bell peppers. Cook for 5 to 10 minutes or until the beef is cooked through and the peppers and onions are soft.
2. Spoon the mixture into the lettuce cups and sprinkle cheese on top. Sprinkle with fresh cilantro! Serve hot!

Prep Time: 10 Minutes

Cook Time: 25 Minutes

Servings: 4

Ingredients

- 1 garlic clove crushed
- 1 onion medium, coarsely chopped
- 1 ginger root 2 inch piece, crushed
- 1 tablespoon olive oil
- 10 ounces beef sliced into strips, sirloin or flank will work great
- 10 ounces broccoli florets
- 1 bell pepper seeded and sliced
- 1/4 cup soy sauce lite (low-sodium), optional tamari or coconut aminos
- 1/2 teaspoon honey
- 3 tablespoons lemon juice fresh
- 1/4 teaspoon ground black pepper
- 1/2 cup water divided
- 1 tablespoon cornstarch or arrowroot

Instructions

1. Over medium heat, in a wok or saucepan with olive oil, sauté the garlic, ginger and onion for 3 minutes. Add the beef and cook for 5 minutes. Add the broccoli and bell pepper.
2. In a small bowl, mix the soy sauce, honey, lemon, and ground pepper. Adjust to taste.
3. In another small bowl, mix the starch and half of the water. Set aside.
4. Pour the soy sauce mixture in the wok then add the remaining half of the water. Cook for 10 - 15 minutes or until the vegetables are cooked through but still crispy. Pour the cornstarch mixture and cook until the sauce is thick. Serve with steamed brown rice or quinoa.

Prep Time: 10 Minutes

Cook Time: 15 Minutes

Servings: 6

Ingredients

- 1 1/2 cups vegetable broth
- 8 ounces cream cheese fat-free, diced into medium-sized cubes
- 6 cups baby spinach
- 1 pound whole-grain spaghetti cooked
- 1/2 cup mozzarella cheese part-skim, low-fat, shredded

Instructions

1. In a large skillet, bring the vegetable broth to a simmer. Add the cream cheese one cube at a time and whisk until smooth. Gently stir in the spinach and cook until spinach is wilted. Stir often to prevent the sauce from burning.

2. Stir in the cooked pasta and toss to coat in the sauce.
    Top with the shredded mozzarella and cover until the
    cheese has melted. Serve and enjoy!

Prep Time: 10 Minutes

Cook Time: 35 Minutes

Servings: 8

Ingredients

- 2 teaspoons olive oil
- 1 yellow onion diced small
- 2 garlic cloves minced
- 1 red bell pepper diced small
- 1 teaspoon ground cumin
- 1 teaspoon smoked paprika
- 1/2 teaspoon ground black pepper
- 1 teaspoon kosher salt
- 1/2 teaspoon ground oregano
- 4 cups black beans cooked (is using canned, rinse well)
- 15 ounces diced tomatoes can
- 4 cups vegetable broth
- 1 avocado peeled, pit removed and diced small
- 1/4 cup cilantro fresh, chopped
- 1 lime cut into wedges

Instructions

1. In a large soup pot, heat the olive oil on medium heat. Once hot, add the onion, garlic, and bell pepper. Cook for about 5 minutes or until the onions just being to soften. Stir in the cumin, paprika, pepper, salt, and oregano. Cook for another minute.
2. Stir in the beans, tomatoes and vegetable broth. Bring to a simmer and simmer for 30 minutes, uncovered.
3. Ladle into serving bowls and top with diced avocado and cilantro. Squeeze one lime wedge over each bowl of soup. Enjoy!

Prep Time: 15 Minutes

Cook Time: 4hrs 30 Minutes

Servings: 6

Ingredients

- 1 yellow onion chopped small
- 1 green bell pepper chopped small
- 2 celery stalks chopped small
- 2 carrots large, peeled and chopped small
- 4 garlic cloves minced
- 3 cups vegetable broth
- 30 ounces diced tomatoes cans
- 30 ounces kidney beans cans, rinsed and drained
- 1 1/2 cups asparagus chopped or optional okra for a more traditional Gumbo
- 1 1/2 cups mushrooms cut into quarters
- 2 tablespoons soy sauce
- 2 tablespoons cajun seasoning
- 1/4 teaspoon kosher salt
- 1/2 teaspoon dried thyme not ground
- 2 tablespoons tomato paste

- 2 cups brown rice cooked

- 1/4 cup parsley fresh, chopped

Instructions

1. Combine all ingredients, except tomato paste, rice, and parsley, in a slow cooker. Cook on low for 8 hours or high for 4 hours.

2. Stir in the tomato paste and cook for 30 minutes on high or until thickened.

3. Spoon rice into serving bowls, ladle gumbo over rice and sprinkle parsley on top. Serve and enjoy!

Prep Time: 10 Minutes

Cook Time: 30 Minutes

Servings: 6

Ingredients

Borscht:

- 1 carrot large
- 1/2 pound celery root
- 1 red onion medium
- 1 zucchini medium
- 1 tomato medium
- 1/2 red bell pepper large
- 6 ounces red cabbage small
- 1/2 pound beets medium
- 3 cups vegetable broth plus additional broth for liquid saute
- 1 lemon

Salt and pepper to taste:

- 1/4 cup parsley fresh, chopped (optional)
- Tofu Sour Cream (optional)

- 12 ounces silken tofu extra-firm, drained

- 1 tablespoon lemon juice

- 1 tablespoon red wine vinegar

- Salt to taste

Instructions

Borscht:

1. Peel and wash the vegetables.
2. Grate the carrots, celery root, zucchini, red cabbage, and beets using a food processor or medium grate.
3. Chop the onion, tomato, and bell pepper into 1/2 inch cubes or smaller.
4. Liquid sauté the grated and chopped vegetables in pan for 3 to 5 minutes: Heat several tablespoons of vegetable broth in a pan over medium-high heat until bubbling, then add veggies and liquid sauté until just al dente, just as you would with oil, frequently deglazing pan with wooden spatula and additional broth if it evaporates.
5. Heat 3 cups vegetable broth in large pot until boiling, then reduce heat to simmer.

6. Add sautéed veggies to broth and simmer for 20 to 25 minutes, adding salt and pepper to taste, and simmer until veggies are tender.

7. Squeeze in the juice of 1 lemon to taste for traditional sour flavor.

8. Tofu Sour Cream (optional)

9. Combine all ingredients in high-speed blender then puree until smooth and creamy.

10. Chill before serving.

11. Store in refrigerator in a sealed container and use within 2 weeks.

12. Optional: serve as a garnish, finely chopped parsley and a dollop of freshly made tofu sour cream

Prep Time: 1hr 30 Minutes

Cook Time: 00 Minutes

Servings: 8

Ingredients

- 28 ounces tofu blocks, extra-firm, organic
- 3 pounds yukon gold potatoes
- 1 onion medium, roughly chopped
- 8 ounces mushrooms package, sliced
- 2 carrots large, or 3 medium
- 1/2 cup green beans fresh or frozen
- 10 ounces peas package, frozen
- 1/2 cup sweet corn kernels fresh or frozen
- 2 tablespoons Italian seasoning or equal blend of basil, marjoram, oregano, rosemary and thyme
- 1 tablespoon dried oregano
- 3 Not-Chick'n Cubes
- 1 tablespoon arrowroot powder or cornstarch
- salt and black pepper to taste
- 1 1/2 cups vegetable broth or as needed

Instructions

1. Press water out of tofu blocks using a tofu press or alternative method, then slice blocks sideways and lengthwise into 4-5 planks, and then cut planks into 1/2" cubes.

2. Boil whole potatoes or steam until soft and easily pierced with a fork. Drain water and mash potatoes thoroughly by hand, or using a mixer, until smooth and all lumps are removed, adding vegetable broth as needed. The mashed potatoes should be able to spread easily over the pie. Cover and set aside.

3. Preheat oven to 350.

4. Add 1/3 cup vegetable broth to a non-stick sauté pan, then sauté onions and mushrooms over medium-high heat until onions are semi-translucent, replenishing vegetable broth and deglazing pan as needed.

5. Add salt, pepper, and seasonings. Add remainder of vegetables and sauté for about 5 minutes, or until al dente. When finished, add cooked vegetables to the deep dish pan.

6. Add 1/2 cup of vegetable broth to the same non-stick pan over medium-high heat until bubbling. Add tofu cubes and sauté until browned, replenishing vegetable broth and deglazing pan as the broth evaporates.

7. When browned, add tofu cubes and toss with the cooked vegetables.

8. Add 4 cups water to the same non-stick sauté pan, then add 3 Not-Chick'n Cubes to water, add arrowroot powder or cornstarch, and bring to a boil for 5 minutes to reduce a bit. Add this broth to the deep dish pan.

9. Add additional salt and pepper to taste. Spread mashed potatoes evenly over the vegetable broth mixture. Mashed potato layer should be at least 1-inch thick.

10. Bake mixture uncovered for one hour.

11. If desired, set oven to broil or increase oven temperature to 450 degrees for 10 minutes to crisp the top of the mashed potatoes.

Prep Time: 10 Minutes

Cook Time: 20 Minutes

Servings: 4

Ingredients

- 2 cups broccoli cut into small florets
- 1/4 cup red onion chopped small
- 3 cloves garlic minced
- 2 cups mushrooms sliced
- 1/4 teaspoon crushed red pepper (optional)
- 2 teaspoons ginger fresh, grated
- 1/4 cup vegetable broth optional water
- 1/2 cup carrot shredded
- 1/4 cup cashews optional water chestnuts
- 2 tablespoons rice wine vinegar
- 2 tablespoons soy sauce low-sodium
- 1 tablespoon coconut sugar optional
- 1 tablespoon sesame seeds

Instructions

1. In a large skillet on high heat, add the broccoli, onion, garlic, mushrooms, red pepper, ginger, and water. Cook, stirring often until broccoli is soft and onions are translucent. Add broth and more as needed to prevent the vegetables from sticking.

2. Stir in the carrot, cashews, vinegar, soy sauce, and coconut sugar. Stir well and simmer for about 2 minutes. Sprinkle with sesame seeds. Serve alone or on top of quinoa or brown rice.

Prep Time: 00 Minutes

Cook Time: 00 Minutes

Servings: 6

Ingredients

- 1/2 cup quinoa dry, pre-rinsed
- 1 cup water
- 1 cup green lentils cooked, well drained
- 1/4 cup red bell pepper diced
- 1/2 cup onion diced
- 2 garlic cloves minced
- 1/2 cup gluten free bread crumbs or whole wheat panko bread crumbs (add additional bread crumbs if the meatballs need to be firmer and aren't holding together well)
- 1/4 cup parmesan freshly grated
- 1 tablespoon parsley leaves flat, freshly chopped
- 1 tablespoon oregano freshly chopped
- 1/2 teaspoon black pepper freshly ground
- Sea salt to taste
- 1/4 teaspoon cayenne pepper

- 1 egg white (for vegan add 2-3 teaspoons water)
- 3 tablespoons olive oil

Instructions

1. Add pre-rinsed quinoa and water to a medium pot, cover, bring to a boil. Reduce heat to a simmer and continue cooking 15 minutes or until water is completely absorbed. In the meantime, in a large non-stick skillet add 1 tablespoon olive oil, heat to medium-low and sauté diced onions and bell pepper until tender about 4 minutes, add garlic, parsley and oregano and sauté one additional minute.

2. Remove quinoa from heat and allow to rest 10 minutes. Press down on quinoa with a paper towel to remove any remaining water.

3. In a large mixing bowl combine sautéed onion, garlic, parsley and oregano along with remaining ingredients, except oil. Use either a potato masher or fork and mash the ingredients until the lentils are well mashed. Using your hands, shape into 1 ½ " (meatless) meatballs, place in a large bowl, cover and refrigerate until chilled, about 2 hours.

4. Add remaining 2 tablespoons oil to a large non-stick skillet, heat to medium-low and add quinoa (meatless) meatballs. Brown meatballs, turn over and brown on the other side. Cook until browned and heated through, about 16 minutes. Remove from skillet and drain on a paper towel.

5. If you plan to serve these (meatless) meatballs with marinara, add to the marinara sauce, gently turn to coat. Simmer until hot and serve over pasta.

6. These are a perfect food to eat prior to working out as they provide complex carbohydrates for energy and protein for building muscles. When on hand, I'll have a few before a workout.

7. TIP: For a vegan version, use vegan egg replacer or 1 tbsp of flax meal mixed with 3 tbsp water rather than the 2-3 teaspoons straight water.

Prep Time: 10 Minutes

Cook Time: 10 Minutes

Servings: 4

Ingredients

- 1 tablespoon olive oil
- 1 red onion sliced thin
- 1 green bell pepper sliced thin
- 1/2 cup carrots peeled and shredded
- 1 cup black beans cooked (if using canned, drained and rinsed)
- 1 teaspoon ground cumin
- 1 tablespoon chili powder
- 1/2 teaspoon kosher salt
- 2 cups kale stems removed and chopped
- 1 jalapeno pepper minced
- 1/4 cup cilantro fresh, chopped
- 4 whole-wheat flour tortillas

Instructions

1. In a large skillet, heat the olive oil on medium heat.
    Once hot, add the onion, bell pepper, and carrot. Cook
    just until the onion begins to turn translucent, about 4
    minutes. Add the black beans, cumin, chili powder,
    salt, kale, and jalapeno. Cook for another 5 minutes or
    until the beans are hot. Stir in the cilantro.

2. Lay the flour tortillas on a flat surface and divide the
    vegetable mixture evenly between the tortillas in the
    center of each. Fold in the sides of the tortillas and roll
    each into a burrito shape. Cut in half and serve.

Prep Time: 10 Minutes

Cook Time: 30 Minutes

Servings: 6

Ingredients

- 1 tablespoon olive oil
- 1 onion medium, diced
- 30 ounces black beans cans, drained
- 1 cup dry quinoa rinsed
- 1/2 cup dry green lentils rinsed (note: green lentils are packed with fiber)
- 3 tablespoons chili powder heaping tablespoons
- 1 teaspoon cumin
- 1/2 teaspoon black pepper
- 1 teaspoon sea salt more or less to taste
- 4 ounces diced green chiles can
- 6 ounces tomato paste can
- 15 ounces diced tomatoes can, with juice
- 1 cup tomato juice
- 4 cups water more or less depending on desired thickness

Instructions

1. In a large pot add oil and onions, over medium-low heat, saute until onions are tender, about 6 minutes.
2. Add the remaining ingredients, stir, and bring to a boil. Reduce heat to a low-boil, cover but leave the lid slightly ajar.
3. Cook chili for 30 minutes or until lentils are tender.
4. Garnish with sour cream and green onions.

Prep Time: 5 Minutes

Cook Time: 20 Minutes

Servings: 4

Ingredients

For the Potato:

- 1 cup water
- 2 sweet potatoes large, washed well
- 3 tablespoons coconut butter

For the Filling:

- 1/2 tablespoon extra-virgin olive oil
- 4 cups baby spinach
- 1/4 cup walnuts slightly crushed
- 1/4 cup raisins

Instructions

For the Potato:

1. Place steamer basket in Instant Pot and add 1 cup water. Using a fork, puncture the potatoes about four times and place the sweet potatoes on top of the steamer basket. Cover and check to be sure the vent is set in the "sealed" position.

2. Press the "steam" button and set the time for 15 minutes. The Instant Pot will begin to preheat. Once ready, the Instant Pot will begin cooking the potatoes for the designated time.

3. When time is completed, wait 5 minutes and then carefully vent the instant pot and remove lid. Cut each sweet potato in half and top each half with coconut butter and top with filling.

For the filling:

1. On a medium skillet, heat olive oil on medium heat. Once hot, add spinach and cook just until the spinach is wilted. Add walnuts and raisins and lightly cook for about 2 minutes, or until the walnuts are lightly toasted. Spoon on top of baked sweet potatoes. Serve and enjoy